The Cookbook for Kidney Conditions

Uncover 30 Recipes Tailored for Kidney Disease Patients

By

Heston Brown

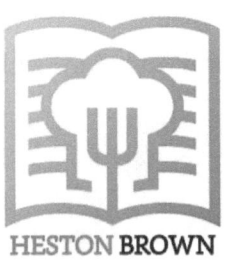

HESTON BROWN

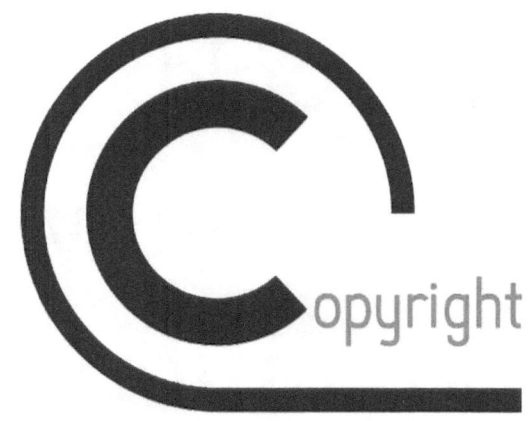

Copyright 2019 Heston Brown

Thank you so much for buying my book! I want to give you a special gift!

Receive a special gift as a thank you for buying my book. Now you will be able to benefit from free and discounted book offers that are sent directly to your inbox every week.

To subscribe simply fill in the box below with your details and start reaping the rewards! A new deal will arrive every day and reminders will be sent so you never miss out. Fill in the box below to subscribe and get started!

https://heston-brown.getresponsepages.com

Subscribe
to our
newsletter

Your Email

Table of Contents

Chapter I - Low Protein Recipes

xxxxxxxxxxxxxxxxxxxxxxxxxxxxxxxxxxxxxxxxxxxxx

Recipe 1: Crab Cakes with Pear Chutney

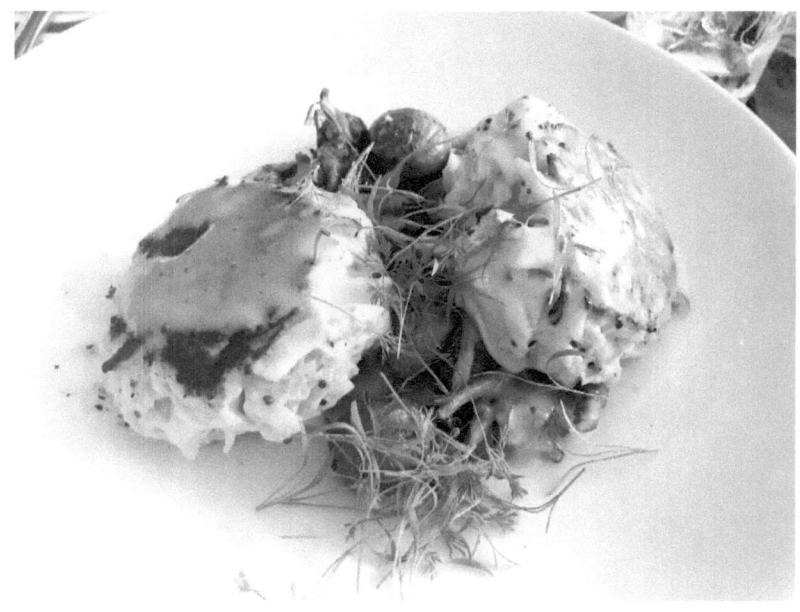

Have you ever tried crab meat? If not, you are missing something really delicious. In this recipe, crab cake or meat is used to make a mouth-watering dish. You can have it alone or combine it with pear chutney, which is a finger-licking sauce. Try it yourself, and you will definitely make it in your next family or friend's get together.

Yield: 2 – 3 persons

Total Prep Time: 10 minutes

Total Cooking Time: 15 minutes

List of Ingredients:

For Crab Cake:

- Crab meat frozen or fresh 120 grams
- · Fresh parsley chopped 1 Tbsp.
- Garlic chopped 1 clove
- Red pepper diced ¼ cup
- Chopped green onion 1 onion
- Egg 1
- Low sodium soya sauce ½ tsp.
- Lemon juice 1 tsp.
- Bread crumbs ¼ cup
- Black pepper freshly grounded ¼ tsp. or to taste
- Vegetable oil to coat the bottom of pan

For Pear Chutney:

- Olive oil 1 Tbsp.
- Red onion chopped 1/3 cup
- Brown sugar 2 Tbsp.
- Cider vinegar 3 Tbsp.
- Black pepper powder ¼ tsp.
- Sage chopped 2 tsp.
- Mustard seed ½ tsp.
- Pears chopped 2 cups (2 medium pears)

xxxxxxxxxxxxxxxxxxxxxxxxxxxxxxxxxxxxxxxxxxxxx

Instructions:

For Crab Cake:

1. In a mixing bowl, add crab meat, parsley, garlic, red pepper, green onion, egg, soya sauce, lemon juice, bread crumbs, and black pepper powder.

2. Mix all the ingredients well.

3. Divide this mixture in eight equal parts.

4. Form crab cakes with the help of your hand, squeeze all the excess liquid.

5. Take a frying pan, add enough vegetable oil to coat the bottom of the pan and heat over medium heat.

6. Sauté the cakes on each side for two minutes or until golden brown.

7. Serve immediately after cooking.

8. Garnish with a lemon slice and sprinkle some chopped parsley.

9. Serve with pears chutney.

For Pear Chutney:

1. Heat olive oil in a pan, sauté red onion until soft.

2. Add brown sugar, cider vinegar, black pepper, chopped sage, mustard seeds, and pears.

3. Cook until the pears are tender.

4. Let it cool.

5. Add the pear mixture in a blender.

6. Blend until smooth.

7. Serve with crab cakes.

8. Reserve the remaining chutney in an airtight jar and keep it in refrigerator.

Recipe 2: Red Soup with Garlic Croutons

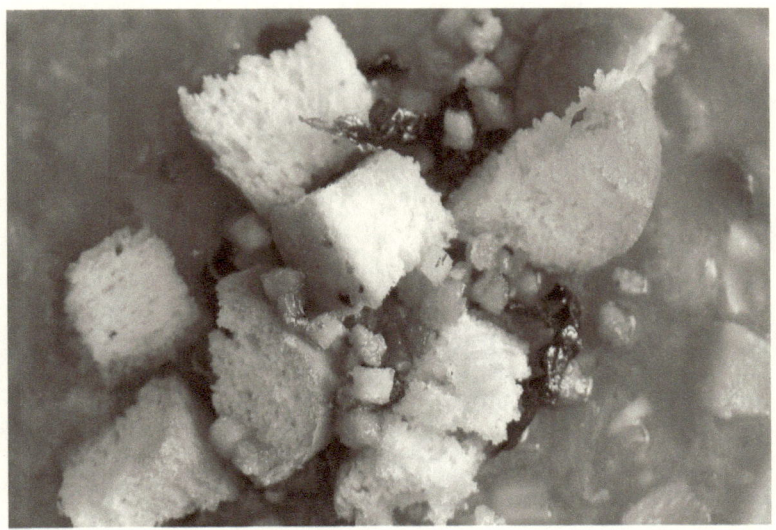

If you are a soup lover, you should try this soup. It is very tasty, easy to make and a unique recipe. Use of olive oil instead of ordinary cooking oil, makes it safe for you. You can have this soup in lunch or in winter evenings.

List of Ingredients:

Yield: 2 – 3 persons

Total Prep Time: 15 minutes

Total Cooking Time: 20 minutes

For Red Soup:

- Red peppers roasted 5 large (10 oz. jar)
- Water 5 cups
- Yellow onion small chopped 2 small onions
- Garlic 5 cloves
- Olive oil 1 Tbsp.
- Fresh basil ½ cup
- Black pepper freshly grounded ½ tsp.
- Hot sauce ¼ tsp.

For Garlic croutons:

- Bread slices 2 thick slices
- Olive oil 4 Tbsp.
- Minced garlic 2 cloves

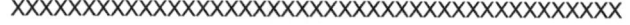

xxxxxxxxxxxxxxxxxxxxxxxxxxxxxxxxxxxxxxxxxxxxxx

Instructions:

1. First prepare garlic croutons, trim bread crust and cut the bread in to small cubes.

2. Take a bowl and add olive oil, bread cubes, and minced garlic and toss them.

3. Spread them on a baking tray.

4. Cook in a preheated oven on 400 degrees for 10 minutes or until golden brown.

5. For soup, take a pan and sauté garlic, onion, and olive oil until aromatic and soft.

6. In a blender, add peppers, garlic, onion, basil, hot sauce, black pepper and make smooth paste.

7. Add water slowly to pepper puree until desired consistency.

8. Can be served hot or chilled, in both ways with garlic croutons.

Recipe 3: Cranberry Glaze Torte

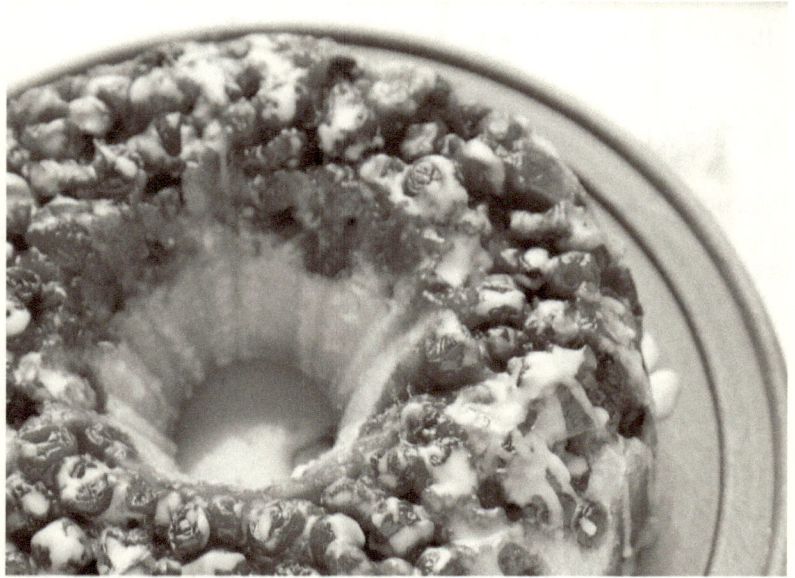

This is a very delicious and easy to make recipe of torte. Being a person with kidney problem doesn't mean that you cannot eat something sweet. Try out this torte. It's low in protein. Cranberry is a very safe way to soothe your sweet cravings

Yield: 5 – 6

Total Prep Time: 15 minutes

Total Cooking Time: 15 minutes

Chilling Time: 4 hours

List of Ingredients:

- Graham crackers crumbs 1 ½ cup
- Unsalted pecans chopped ¼ cup
- SPLENDA sweetener 1 ¾ cup
- Non hydrogenated margarine ½ cup (unsalted and melted)
- Ground fresh cranberries 1 ½ cup
- Egg whites 2
- Frozen apple juice concentrate 1 Tbsp. thawed
- Vanilla extract 1 tsp.
- Light Coolwhip whipped topping 1 L thawed

For Cranberry Glaze:

- SPLENDA sweetener ¼ cup
- White granulated sugar ¼ cup
- Corn starch 1 Tbsp.
- Fresh cranberries ¾ cup
- Water ¾ cup

XX

Instructions:

1. First preheat oven to 375 F.

2. In a large bowl, combine pecans, graham crackers crumb, ¾ cup of Splenda, and margarine mix well.

3. Take an 8 inch spring-form pan and add the mixture of crumbs and pecans in it, press into the bottom and sides of the pan.

4. Bake the crust for 6 to 8 minutes or until light brown.

5. Let it cool.

6. In another bowl, combine 1 cup Splenda and cranberries.

7. Let stand for 5 minutes.

8. Add apple juice, egg whites, and vanilla, beat on low speed until frothy.

9. Then beat on high speed for 6 to 8 minutes until stiff peaks form.

10. Whip coolwhip into the berries mixture.

11. Pour the mixture into the prepared crust.

12. Freeze for at least 4 hours or until firm.

13. To prepare the glaze combine together the Splenda, granulated sugar, and corn starch in a pan.

14. Stir in water and the cranberries.

15. Stir and cook until bubbly.

16. Stir occasionally; continue to cook until the cranberry skins pop.

17. Cook to room temperature.

18. Do not chill because the sauce will become cloudy or the sauce may crystallize.

19. To serve tort take a serving plate remove the torte from the pan and place on plate.

20. Spoon the cranberry glaze on top.

Recipe 4: Zucchini with Daiya Cheese Lasagna

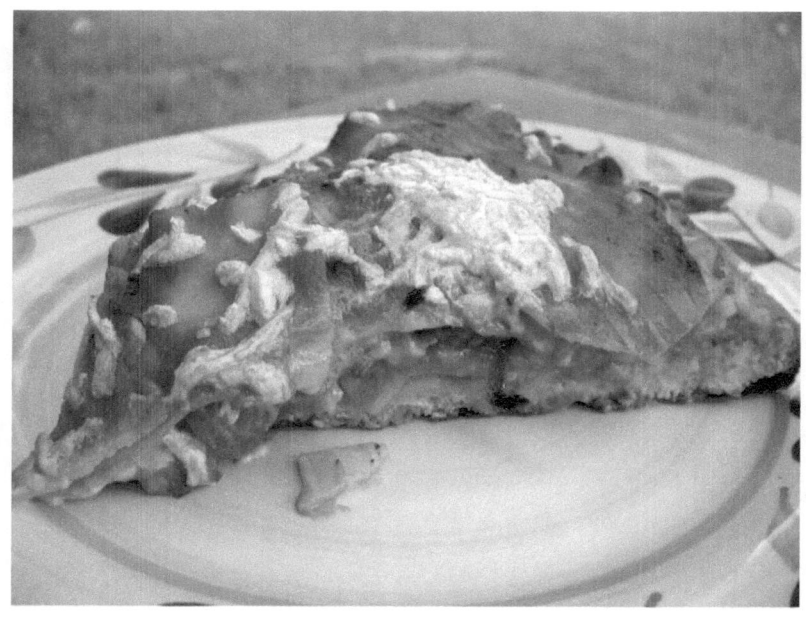

Zucchini is vegetable with lots of health benefits. It helps in regulating your metabolic system, helps in regulating your blood pressure, etc. It is important to include this beneficial vegetable in your diet, and use it regularly. This lasagna recipe is quick, easy, and delicious. Addition of cheese make it attractive for kids as well.

Yield: 3 persons

Total Prep Time: 20 minutes

Total Cooking Time:20 minutes

List of Ingredients:

- Zucchini peeled and sliced 4 small
- Daiya mozzarella cheese shredded ¾ cup (6 oz.)
- Parmesan cheese grated 2 Tbsp. (2 oz.)
- Olive oil 2 Tbsp.
- Minced garlic 1 clove
- Fresh thyme 3 sprigs
- Pepper   ¼ tsp. or to taste

xxxxxxxxxxxxxxxxxxxxxxxxxxxxxxxxxxxxxxxxxxxxxx

Instructions:

1. Preheat your oven to 350 degree.

2. Cut zucchini into slices by using a mandolin slicer.

3. Season with pepper.

4. Heat olive oil in a frying pan, add zucchini slices and minced garlic in it.

5. Sauté for 4 to 5 minutes or until soften.

6. Grease a medium sized baking pan, layer zucchini slices in it and top it with layer of shredded Daiya mozzarella cheese.

7. Repeat the layers, ending with a top layer of zucchini slices (to create beauty woven zucchini slices into a crisscross formation)

8. Lastly top with grated parmesan cheese and sprinkle fresh thyme.

9. Place on center rack of your oven and cook for 15 minutes or until topping is golden brown color.

Recipe 5: Tortilla Pizza with Shrimps and Basil

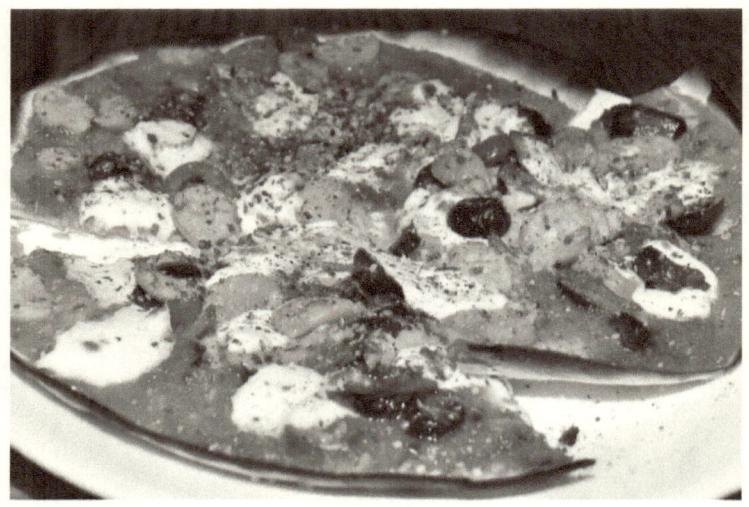

Who loves pizza? Do you love it? I love pizza so much and cannot quit it at any cost. Well! Here is a very nutritious recipe of tortilla pizzas. This pizza is healthy, nutritious, and delicious as well. It is a low protein dish, and it is safe for a kidney patient, whose protein intake is restricted. You can make it for your lunch, or if you are a true pizza lover, you can have it as evening snack too.

Yield: 1 -2

Total Prep Time: 25 minutes

Total Cooking Time: 15 minutes

List of Ingredients:

For the tortilla pizza:

- Flour tortillas 2
- Shrimps 8 large (peeled, tail removed, and deveined)
- Vidalia onion sliced ¼ cup
- Basil leaves torn or roughly chopped 6 leaves
- Grated mozzarella cheese ½ cup

For pesto:

- Red pepper roasted 1
- ·Garlic   1 clove
- Lemon juice 1 Tbsp.
- Extra virgin olive oil 1 Tbsp.
- Freshly grounded black pepper 1/8 tsp.
- Parmesan cheese grated 1 tsp.

xxx

Instructions:

1. To make pesto, add red pepper, garlic, lemon juice, olive oil, black pepper, and parmesan cheese to blender and blend well until smooth.

2. Preheat oven to 400 F.

3. Place the oven rack in middle of the oven.

4. Slice shrimps in half lengthwise.

5. Grease a cookie sheet.

6. Place flour tortillas on it divide the pesto between the two tortillas.

7. Spread to cover the tortilla surface.

8. Add the basil and onion on it.

9. Evenly sprinkle mozzarella cheese on tortillas.

10. Place shrimps on top of the pizzas.

11. Bake for 10 minutes or until shrimps turn pink in color, tortillas crisp and turn nice golden brown.

12. Take out from oven and rest them for 2 to 3 minutes then serve.

Recipe 6: Rice Salad with Salmon and French Dressing

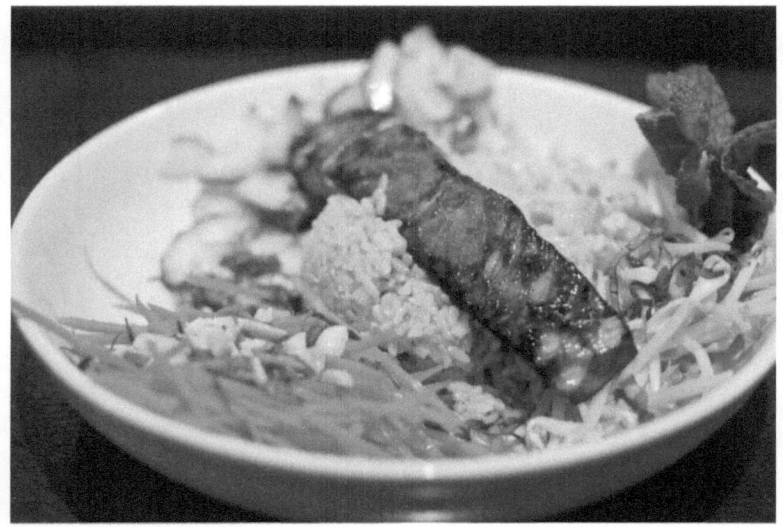

Rice salad is a nutritious and tasty dish. With salmon, vegetables, and French dressing, it is a perfect meal for your lunch. You can also use it as a side dish in your dinner. You can give it to your kids as well, and they will love it.

Yield: 4 persons

Total Prep Time: 1 hour 15 minutes

Total Cooking Time: 20 minutes

List of Ingredients:

- Rice uncooked ½ cup
- Water 2 cups
- French dressing ¼ cup (50 ml)
- Pepper ¼ tsp. (1gm)
- Onion finely chopped 1 Tbsp.
- Cucumber sliced ½ cup
- Horseradish 1 tsp.
- Celery seed ½ tsp. (2gm)
- Chopped celery ½ cup
- Egg cooked chopped 1 egg
- Low sodium salmon drained ½ cup

xxxxxxxxxxxxxxxxxxxxxxxxxxxxxxxxxxxxxxxxxxx

Instructions:

1. Heat a sauce pan, add 2 cups water, cover and bring it to boil.

2. Add rice and simmer on medium low heat to cook rice for 10 to 15 minutes.

3. Remove cooked rice from pan, let sit covered for 10 minutes.

4. To the hot cooked rice, add French dressing and toss.

5. Cool rice to room temperature, and then add pepper, onion, cucumber, horseradish, celery seed, chopped celery, chopped egg, and low sodium drained salmon.

6. Now mix lightly, cover and keep in refrigerator.

7. Chill this rice salad at least one hour before serving.

Recipe 7: Stir Fry Tofu and Vegetables with Rice

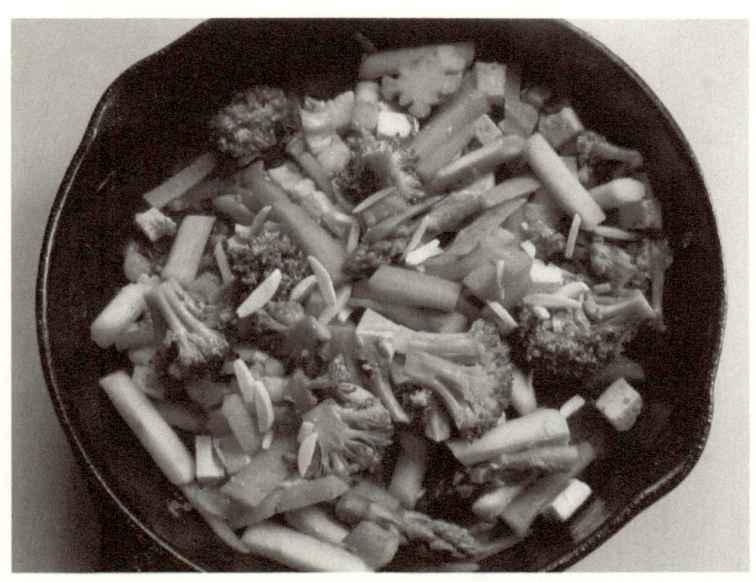

Tofu is a good source of calcium, all eight essential amino acids, Vitamin B1, selenium, and manganese. This dish is best for dinner. If you are bored of eating the regular food all week long, this dish is for you. This recipe serves food with low protein content. You can also add yellow or red bell pepper to make your dish colorful.

Yield: 4 -5

Total Prep Time: 25 minutes

Total Cooking Time: 15 minutes

List of Ingredients:

- Long grain rice uncooked 1 cup
- Hoisin sauce 2 ½ Tbsp. (without potassium preservative)
- Fresh lime juice 2 Tbsp.
- Medium firm tofu 1 package (prepared with calcium sulfate)
- Canola oil 1 Tbsp.
- Carrot 1 medium size
- Bell pepper 1 medium size
- Grated fresh ginger 1 Tbsp.
- Bean sprouts 2 cups
- Scallions thinly sliced 4
- Roasted peanuts roughly chopped 2 Tbsp.
- Fresh cilantro chopped ¼ cup

xxxxxxxxxxxxxxxxxxxxxxxxxxxxxxxxxxxxxxxxxxxx

Instructions:

1. Cut tofu into ½ inch cubes.

2. Cut carrot in thin strips.

3. Cut bell pepper in thin slices.

4. First cook rice and set aside.

5. Whisk hoisin sauce and lime juice together.

6. Heat the oil in a large wok over medium high heat.

7. Add the ginger, carrot, and bell pepper and cook.

8. Continue stirring for 2 minutes.

9. Now add bean sprouts and tofu, stir continuously for 3 to 4 minutes or until the vegetables are slightly tender.

10. Bean sprouts should be fully cooked.

11. Add hoisin sauce mixture in it, toss the vegetables with sauce.

12. Serve these stir fry vegetables over rice.

13. Sprinkle chopped peanuts, scallions, and cilantro on top and serve hot.

Recipe 8: Classic Blueberry Pancakes

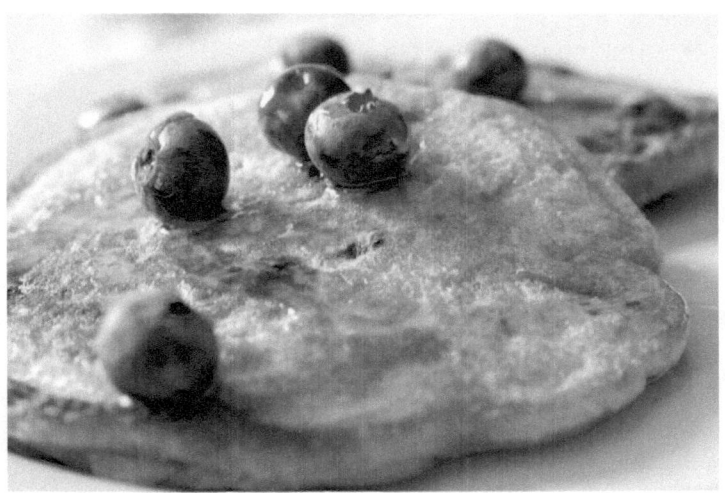

This is a classic pancake recipe that is perfect for your breakfast. These blueberry pancakes are a healthy enough to start your day and stay active. Kids, adults all like them equally. You can also use butter, if you don't have margarine or you don't want to use it. Make sure butter is unsalted as it may affect the taste and texture of pancakes.

Yield: 4 – 5 persons

Total Prep Time: 15 minutes

Total Cooking Time: 10 minutes

List of Ingredients:

- All-purpose flour sifted 1 ½ cup

- Baking powder 2 tsp.

- Sugar 3 Tbsp.

- Butter milk 1 cup

- Unsalted margarine melted 2 Tbsp.

- Slightly beaten eggs 2

- Blueberries canned or frozen rinsed 1 cup

- Vanilla essence 1 drop

- Vegetable oil to grease pan ½ tsp. or as required

xxxxxxxxxxxxxxxxxxxxxxxxxxxxxxxxxxxxxxxxxxxx

Instructions:

1. In a mixing bowl, sift together baking powder, flour, and sugar.

2. Make a well in the center of the sifted ingredients and add butter milk, margarine, eggs, vanilla essence, and blueberries.

3. Start to mix all ingredients from the center and gradually mix in the dry ingredients.

4. Make a smooth batter and begin to cook immediately.

5. Take a 12-inch heavy griddle or skillet and grease it lightly with vegetable oil.

6. Spoon out pancakes using 1/3 cup measuring cup and cook until done.

7. Flip the pancake only one time otherwise they will break.

8. Serve hot.

Recipe 9: Blueberry and Vanilla Muffins

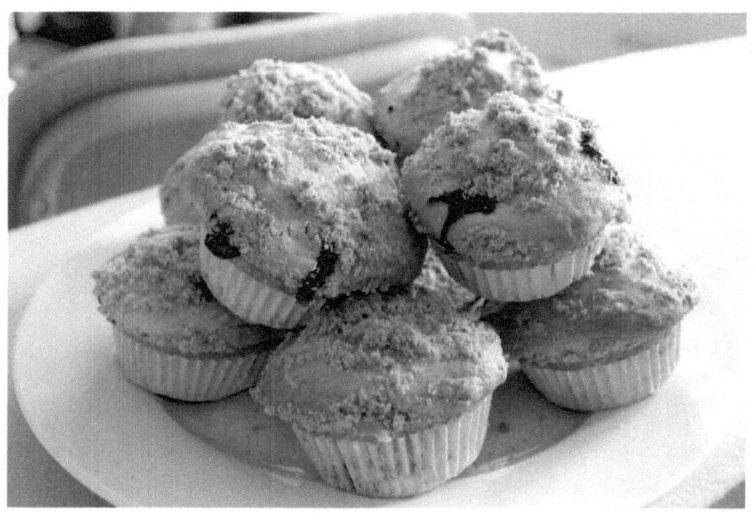

Kids and adults both like muffins. If prepared carefully with healthy ingredients, muffins are very nutritious and fulling. These muffins contain all healthy ingredients. You can use them in your breakfast, or as evening snacks. Kids can take these muffins as snacks to their schools as well. Instead of frozen blueberries, you can also use fresh ones. The good thing about Blueberry and Vanilla muffins is that you can store them for up to one week.

Yield: 5 – 6

Total Prep Time: 20 minutes

Total Cooking Time: 25 minutes

List of Ingredients:

- Sugar 1 cup (250gms)
- Eggs 2
- Oil ½ cup (125 ml)
- Wheat bran (germ removed) 2 cups
- Vanillas extract 2 tsp. (10 ml)
- White flour 2 cups
- Baking powder 4 tsp.
- Baking soda 2 tsp.
- Plain yogurt 2 cups
- Frozen blueberries 1 cup

xxxxxxxxxxxxxxxxxxxxxxxxxxxxxxxxxxxxxxxxxxxxx

Instructions:

1. Place the rack of your oven in middle position and preheat oven to 375 F.

2. In a bowl mix egg, sugar, wheat bran, vanillas extract, and oil.

3. Mix baking soda and yogurt together.

4. Mix white flour, baking powder in another bowl.

5. Now combine all the ingredients with blueberries.

6. Line muffin cups with silicon or paper liners.

7. Scoop into each muffin cup.

8. Bake for 20 to 25 minutes or until insert a toothpick in the middle of muffin and it has come out clean.

9. Let it cool then serve hot or save them in an airtight jar.

Recipe 10: Spicy White Mushroom Pasta

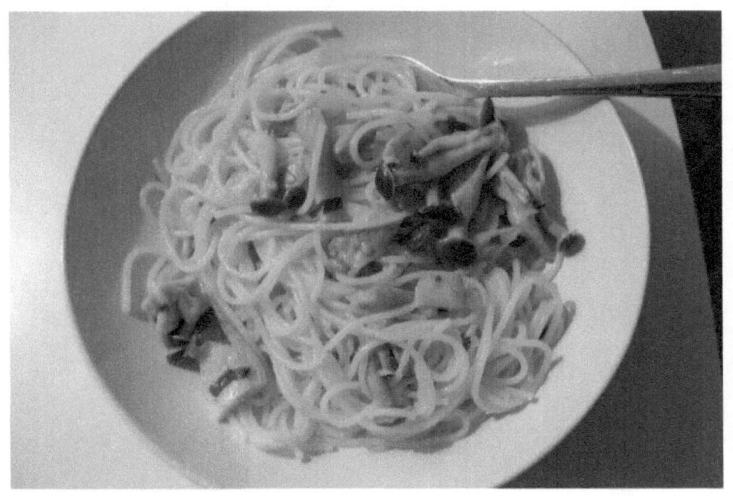

Mushrooms are a great source of fiber, vitamins, protein, and minerals. This single ingredient can add a lot of nutrients to your food. In this recipe, mushrooms are served with pasta, making it more attractive, especially for pasta lovers.

Yield: 2 persons

Total Prep Time: 15 minutes

Total Cooking Time: 40 minutes

List of Ingredients:

- White mushrooms quartered 1 cup
- Boiling water ½ cup
- Dried porcini mushrooms 1 small pack (30gms)
- Olive oil 1/3 cup
- Finely chopped garlic 2 cloves
- Dried hot chili pepper flakes 1 pinch
- Dried sage ¼ tsp.
- Mini Bononcini mozzarella cheese ½ cup
- Fresh parsley chopped 1/3 cup
- Any dried short pasta 2 cups (½ pound)

xxxxxxxxxxxxxxxxxxxxxxxxxxxxxxxxxxxxxxxxxxx

Instructions:

1. Put porcini mushroom in a bowl with ½ cup of hot water to rehydrate.

2. In a pan, bring 3 liters of water to boil to cook pasta. Cook pasta according to the instructions of the packet.

3. Drain the pasta, but do not rinse.

4. To prepare sauce, heat oil in a large pan over medium heat.

5. Add garlic and cook until nice golden brown, then add hot chili pepper flakes in the pan.

6. Now raise the heat to medium high and add white mushrooms.

7. Squeeze the liquid from porcini mushrooms in a bowl and reserve the liquid, chop them and add to the pan.

8. Add the reserved liquid of porcini mushrooms through sieve into the pan.

9. Now add sage and cook for 4 to 6 minutes.

10. Add pasta, toss well into the pan with all the ingredients.

11. Finely add Bononcini mozzarella cheese, parsley and serve hot.

Chapter II - Low Phosphorus Recipes

xxxxxxxxxxxxxxxxxxxxxxxxxxxxxxxxxxxxxxxxxxxxx

Recipe 11: Corn and Egg Potage

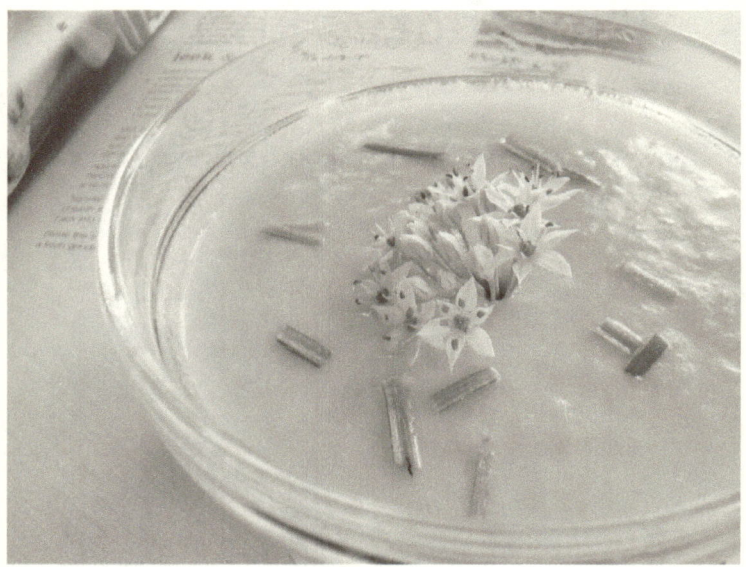

This soup is really delicious and healthy. Corn gives a thick beautiful consistency to the soup. Make sure that you use low sodium soy sauce. You can also use beef broth instead of chicken.

Yield: 5 – 6 persons

Total Prep Time: 15 minutes

Total Cooking Time: 20 minutes

List of Ingredients:

- Unsalted chicken broth 8 cups
- Corn kernels fresh or frozen 2 ¼ cup
- Sugar 1 tsp.
- Black pepper powder 1 pinch
- Corn starch 2 Tbsp.
- Water 2 Tbsp.
- Egg whites lightly beaten 2
- Scallions thinly sliced 4
- Vinegar ½ tsp.
- Low sodium soya sauce ½ tsp.

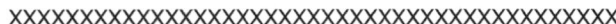

xxxxxxxxxxxxxxxxxxxxxxxxxxxxxxxxxxxxxxxxxxxx

Instructions:

1. Heat a pan and add chicken broth and bring it to boil.

2. Add corn in boiling broth cook for 5 minutes.

3. Strain chicken stock over a heat proof bowl and reserve it.

4. Transfer corns to a blender and blend the corns until smooth.

5. Press the blended corn through a china cap. It will remove any solids.

6. Return chicken stock to a pan add black pepper and bring it to boil.

7. Stir in vinegar, sugar, and soya sauce.

8. Blend corn starch and water in a small bowl.

9. Stir constantly and add cornstarch mixture cook until thickened.

10. Drizzle in egg whites slowly stirring with the spoon in circular motion.

11. Turn off heat add scallions and serve hot.

Recipe 12: Steamed Fish with Bell Peppers

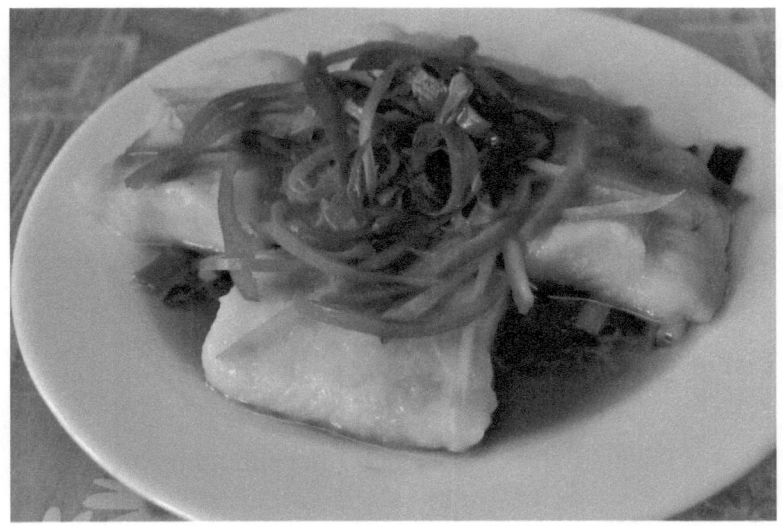

Tilapia is a white and delicious fish with a lot of health benefits. Some of these are:

- Helps in reducing weight
- Boosts your metabolism
- Reduces the risk of chronic heart diseases
- Helps in lowering triglycerides
- Boosts brain power

It is a very easy to make recipe. This dish is low in phosphorus but other ingredients, especially addition of tilapia makes it extremely healthy. Make this colorful dish and give yourself a tasty treat.

Yield: 2 -3 persons

Total Prep Time: 25 minutes

Total Cooking Time: 12 minutes

List of Ingredients:

- Tilapia fish fillets 4 (each fillet should be of 100gms)
- Olive oil 6 Tbsp.
- Sliced green and red peppers ¾ cup
- Sliced onion 1 medium
- Freshly crushed black pepper ¼ tsp.
- Hot pepper sauce 1 tsp.
- Thyme 1 large sprig
- Ketchup 1 Tbsp.
- Lime juice 1 Tbsp.
- Hot water 1 cup

XXX

Instructions:

1. In frying pan heat oil on medium and sauté bell peppers and onion.

2. Add hot pepper sauce, crushed black pepper, ketchup, thyme, and lime juice.

3. Add hot water 1 cup and stir for 2 to 3 minutes.

4. Now place fish fillets in pan and spoon sauce and vegetables over fish.

5. Cover and cook for five minutes.

6. Turn fish fillets gently, cover and cook for five more minutes, or until fully cooked

Recipe 13: Baked Moroccan Chicken

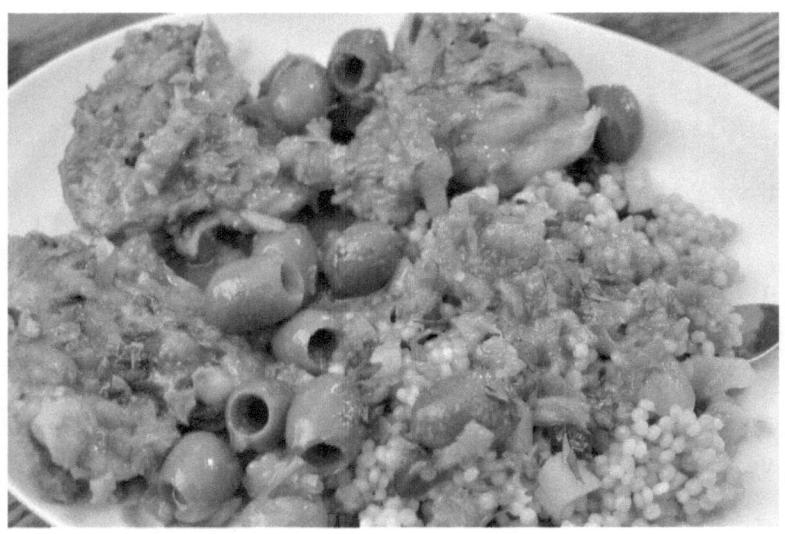

This is a traditional dish of Morocco. It is easy to make. To save time, you can prepare the marinade a day before you want to have this dish. All the ingredients used in this recipe are easily available.

Yield: 4 -5 persons

Total Prep Time: 6 – 12 hours

Total Cooking Time: 45 minutes

List of Ingredients:

- Skinless chicken thighs or breasts 6
- Honey 1/3 cup
- Lemon juice 2 Tbsp.
- Sesame oil 1 tsp.
- Lemon zest ½ tsp.
- Crushed garlic 3 cloves
- Cumin grounded ½ tsp.
- Powdered Onion ¼ tsp.
- Paprika 1 tsp.
- Cinnamon powder ¼ tsp
- Nutmeg ¼ tsp.
- Cayenne pepper ½ tsp.
- Black pepper freshly crushed ¼ tsp.

XXXXXXXXXXXXXXXXXXXXXXXXXXXXXXXXXXXXXXXXXXX

Instructions:

1. Take a big bowl and add honey, lemon juice, lemon zest, sesame oil, crushed garlic, cumin, onion powder, paprika, cinnamon powder, nutmeg, cayenne pepper, and black pepper in it and mix well.

2. Add chicken in the mixture.

3. Keep in the refrigerator for minimum 6 to12 hours or maximum 24 hours.

4. Turn the chicken over every now and then.

5. Foil a baking tray.

6. Place marinated chicken on foil.

7. Pour on top the extra marinade.

8. Bake at 400 degree until fully cooked.

9. Remember to turn the chicken after 25 minutes.

10. Garnish with lemon slices and serve.

Recipe 14: Sweet and Sour Grilled Turkey

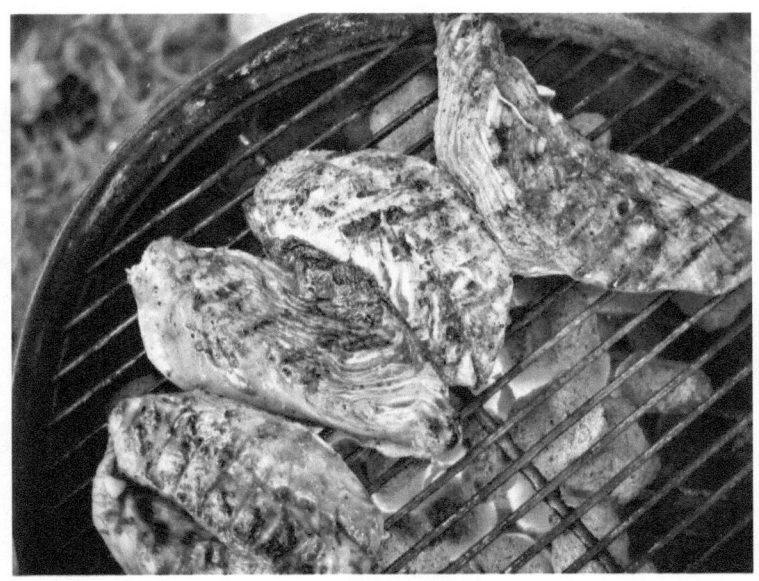

Turkey has very nutritious meat. It is good for overall health, but if your doctor has restricted your protein intake, you should avoid turkey, as it is rich in protein. In this recipe, dried herbs are also used which are rich in anti-oxidants. Although, this dish lies under low phosphorus category, you can prepare this tasty dish for parties or when you invite your friends and family over your place for dinner.

Yield: 4 – 5 persons

Total Prep Time: 3 hours 15 minutes

Total Cooking Time:30 minutes

List of Ingredients:

- Skinless, boneless turkey breast 300gms (2/3 pound)
- Lime juice ½ cup
- ·Liquid honey   2 Tbsp.
- Vegetable oil ¼ cup
- Dried thyme leaves 1 tsp.
- Dried rosemary 1 tsp.
- Black pepper powder ¼ tsp.

xxxxxxxxxxxxxxxxxxxxxxxxxxxxxxxxxxxxxxxxxxxx

Instructions:

1. In a bowl add lime juice, honey, vegetable oil, thyme, rosemary, and black pepper and mix well.

2. Take 2 Tbsp. of this mixture in another small bowl and set aside for basting.

3. Cut turkey breast in thin slices.

4. Now add these thin slices of turkey in marinade and place them in refrigerator for 2 to 3 hours.

5. Grill turkey for 5 minutes each side until fully done.

6. Baste turkey by using marinade set aside while grilling.

7. You can also grill it in your oven, preheat oven broiler on 500 F and cook for 10 minutes per side or until fully cooked.

Recipe 15: Raspberry and Vanilla Mousse

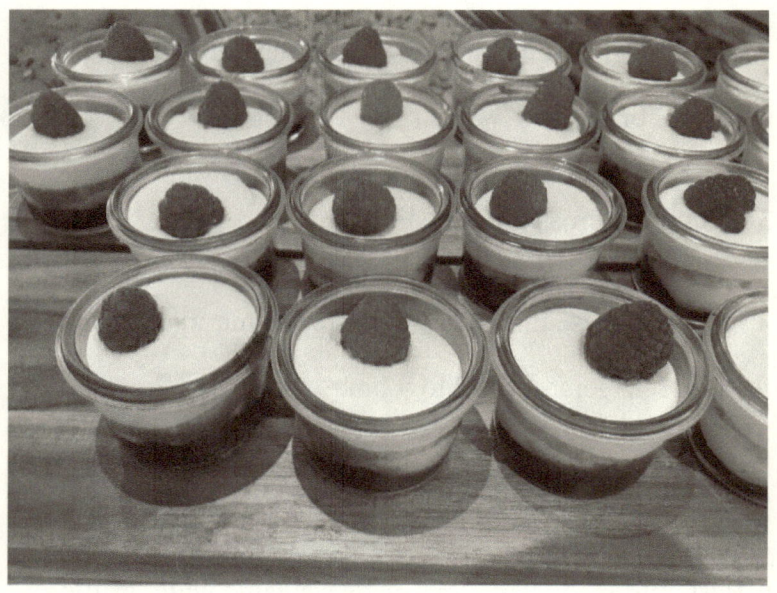

Low phosphorus diet doesn't mean you cannot enjoy any dessert or sweet dish. Raspberry and Vanilla mousses are a good source to satisfy your sweet tooth. In this recipe, you can use both frozen and fresh raspberries, but use of fresh fruit is recommended.

Yield: 6 persons

Total Prep Time: 20 minutes

Chilling Time: 1 – 2 hours

List of Ingredients:

- Light, whipped topping 1 cup
- Cream cheese (room temperature) 1 pack (8 oz.)
- SPLENDA granular (no calorie sweetener) ¾ cup
- Lemon zest finely grated 1 tsp.
- Vanilla extract 1 tsp.
- Raspberries fresh or frozen 1 cup

xxxxxxxxxxxxxxxxxxxxxxxxxxxxxxxxxxxxxxxxxx

Instructions:

1. In a bowl add cream cheese and beat until fluffy.

2. Add ½ cup SPLENDA granular and beat well until melted.

3. Stir in vanilla and lemon zest.

4. Reserve ¼ cup raspberries for garnish.

5. Add ¼ cup SPLENDA granular in remaining raspberries and crush them with the help of fork until SPENDA granular melt and blend with raspberries.

6. In cream cheese mixture fold light, whipped topping.

7. Then quickly but gently fold in crushed raspberry mixture.

8. Into 6 serving glasses spoon mousse.

9. Keep them in refrigerator until chilled.

10. Garnish them with raspberries and serve chilled.

Recipe 16: Stir Fry Shrimps with Apple

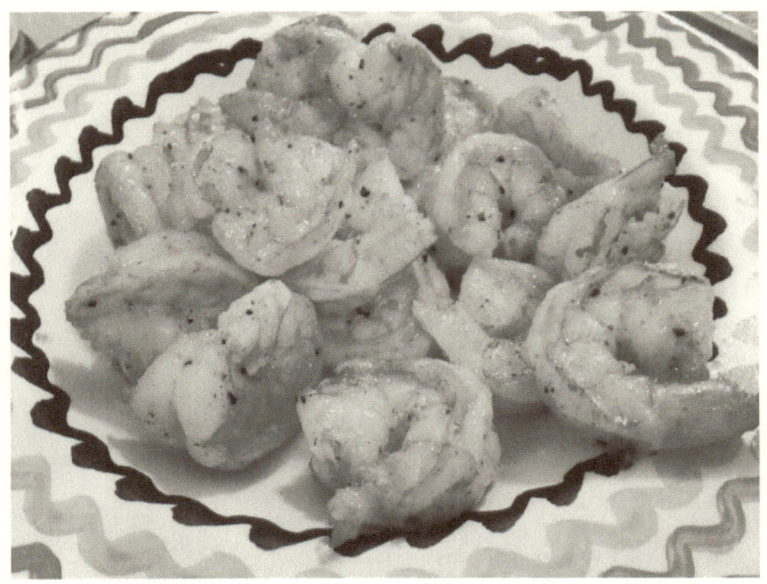

This is another tasty low phosphorus recipe. If you are a sea food lover, this recipe is for you. It is easy to make and delicious at the same time. Kids will also love this recipe, when served with pasta. You can serve with rice as well.

Yield: 3 – 4 persons

Total Prep Time: 1 hour

Total Cooking Time:15 minutes

List of Ingredients:

- Headless shrimps 250gms
- Diced apple ¾
- Diced salary 2 stalks
- Small diced sweet red pepper ½
- Vegetable oil 2 Tbsp.
- Crushed ginger ½ tsp.
- Low sodium soya sauce 1 tsp.
- Cornstarch 2 tsp.
- White pepper ¼ tsp.
- Sugar 1 tsp.
- Cold water 2 Tbsp.
- Red chili flakes ¼ tsp.

xxxxxxxxxxxxxxxxxxxxxxxxxxxxxxxxxxxxxxxxxxx

Instructions:

1. First of all, remove shells, deveined shrimps and wash thoroughly.

2. In a bowl add crushed ginger, soya sauce ½ tsp., cornstarch 1 tsp., white pepper, and red chili flakes, mix well.

3. Marinade shrimps in this mixture for half an hour.

4. Heat 1 Tbsp. oil in a no- stick pan; stir fry the marinade shrimps on medium high flame until they turned pink in color.

5. Remove from the pan.

6. In a non-stick wok heat 1 Tbsp. oil on medium high flame and stir fry celery.

7. Then add diced apples and red peppers and cook for 2 to 3 minutes.

8. Now add shrimps, soya sauce ½ tsp., sugar, cornstarch 1 tsp., and cold water.

9. Keep stirring constantly until sauce thickens.

10. Serve it with boil rice or pasta.

Note: You can store shrimps after marinating them, and use as required. Marinated shrimps can be stored for up to 1 week.

Recipe 17: Baked Chicken with Rice and Sweet Chili Thai Sauce

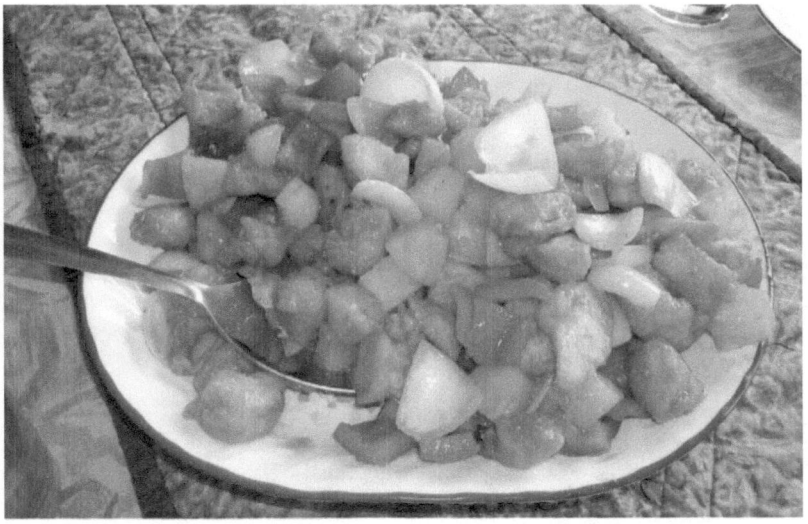

This dish with Thai sauce is delicious. You may have found the preparation time a bit lengthy, but the end result is awesome. Use of little oil makes this dish health friendly as well. You can use spaghetti instead of rice.

Yield: 7 – 8 persons

Total Prep Time: 30 minutes

Total Cooking Time: 40 minutes

List of Ingredients:

For Chicken:

- Skinless boneless chicken breasts 1 pound (4 ½ breasts)
- Egg 1
- Milk 2 Tbsp.
- Flour ¼ cup
- Corn flakes 2 ½ cup
- Garlic powder ½ tsp.
- Ginger powder ¼ tsp.
- Mrs. Dash 1 tsp.
- Chili powder ½ tsp.
- Red pepper flakes ½ tsp.

For the rice:

- Cooked rice 4 cups
- Bean sprouts 1 cup
- Carrot diced 1 ½ cup
- Red pepper ½
- Yellow pepper ½
- Celery chopped 1 cup

For sweet chili Thai sauce:

- Cider vinegar ¾ cup
- Water 1 cup
- Sugar ½ cup
- Ginger 1 tsp.
- Minced garlic 1 tsp.
- Red pepper flakes 2 tsp.
- Ketchup 2 tsp.
- Corn starch 4 tsp.

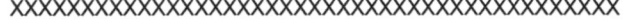

XXXXXXXXXXXXXXXXXXXXXXXXXXXXXXXXXXXXXXXXXX

Instructions:

For the chicken:

1. Add ginger powder and garlic powder to the chicken and leave it for half an hour.

2. In a zip lock bag put cornflakes and crush until small pieces.

3. Beat milk and egg in a bowl.

4. Transfer it in a plate.

5. In a separate plate spread the flour.

6. In a small bowl mix Mrs. Dash, red pepper flakes, and chili powder.

7. Preheat oven on 350 degree.

8. Now take a chicken breast first coat with flour then in milk and egg mixture.

9. Sprinkle the spices mixture evenly over both side of chicken breast.

10. Lastly coat with the crushed cornflakes.

11. Repeat the procedure with remaining chicken breasts.

12. Spray olive oil on a baking sheet and bake the chicken for 45 minutes.

13. Turn the chicken after 20 minutes.

For the Rice:

1. Boil water in a large pot.

2. Add diced carrots and bean sprouts in boiling water and cook for 2 minutes.

3. Then add celery and peppers and cook for 1 more minute. Vegetable should remain crisp, don't overcook them.

4. Strain all the vegetables and mix in cooked rice.

For sweet chili Thai sauce:

1. Boil water.

2. Add cider vinegar, sugar, garlic, ginger, ketchup, and red pepper flakes to the boiling water.

3. Stir and simmer all the ingredients for 5 minutes.

4. While stirring continuously add slowly the cornstarch.

5. Cook until thicken.

Assembling:

Serve the chicken over bed of vegetable rice, and top it with sweet chili Thai sauce.

Recipe 18: Beef Salad with Chili-Lime Vinaigrette Dressing

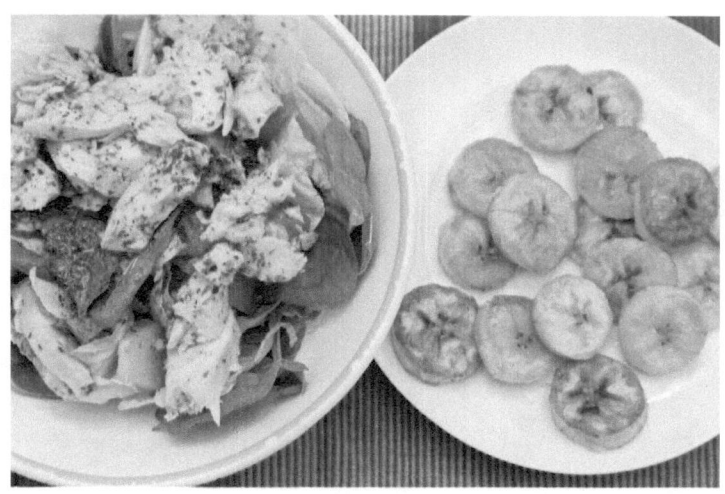

Beef is also known as red meat. Many people don't like to eat beef at all, but it is good to use some amount of beef occasionally. Beef is a vital source of Vitamin B. It also contains heart-healthy fats, same as found in olive oil. Sesame oil is another healthy ingredient of this recipe. It is good for health of heart, bones, teeth, etc.

This recipe is a perfect for your dinner. It is tasty, healthy, and taste-bud satisfying.

Yield: 4 -5 persons

Total Prep Time: 20 minutes

Total Cooking Time: 30 to 40 minutes

List of Ingredients:

- Beef strips 450gms (top sirloin or Flank steak, thinly sliced)
- Sesame oil 1 tsp.
- Asian chili sauce 1 tsp.
- Minced garlic 2 cloves
- Minced ginger 1 Tbsp.
- Fresh lime juice 1 Tbsp.
- Corn starch 1 Tbsp.
- Torn romaine lettuce 8 cups
- Canola oil 4 tsp.
- Grape tomatoes (halved) ½ cup
- Julienned cucumber ½ cup
- Julienned sweet yellow pepper ½ cup
- Julienned red onion ½ cup
- Chili-Lime Vinaigrette dressing
- Grated lime rind 1 tsp.

- Fresh lime juice ¼ cup
- Rice vinegar 2 Tbsp.
- Low sodium soya sauce 1 Tbsp.
- Liquid honey 1 Tbsp.
- Asian chili sauce ¼ tsp.

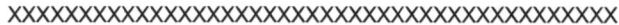

XXXXXXXXXXXXXXXXXXXXXXXXXXXXXXXXXXXXXXXXXXXXX

Instructions:

1. In a bowl combine ginger, garlic, corn starch, sesame oil, lime juice, and chili sauce.

2. Add beef in it toss to coat and leave it for 15 minutes.

3. Discard marinade and keep beef strips.

4. Heat 1 tsp. canola oil on medium high heat in a large fry pan.

5. Stir fry cucumbers, tomatoes, onion, and yellow bell pepper until just wilted.

6. Transfer all these vegetables in a clean bowl.

7. Now heat 3 tsp. of canola oil in same fry pan.

8. Stir fry beef until fully cooked and browned.

9. Also add these beef strips in wilted vegetable bowl.

10. Toss to combine.

11. Take another bowl and add all the ingredients of Chili-Lime Vinaigrette dressing whisk well and cook it in the same fry pan on medium heat.

12. Cook until slightly thickened.

13. Toss romaine with just enough hot Vinaigrette to moisten.

14. Top romaine lettuce with vegetable and beef mixture.

15. Now drizzle remaining Vinaigrette over it.

Recipe 19: Zucchini Chicken Pasta

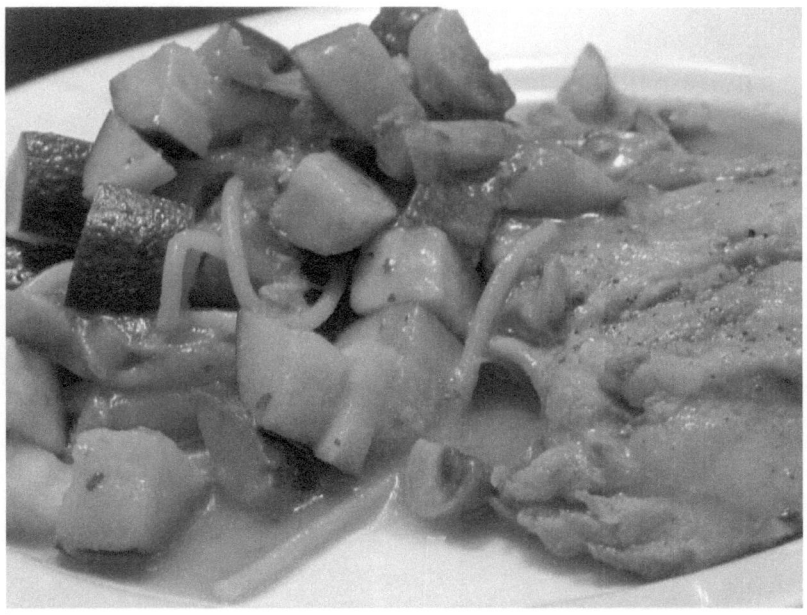

Zucchini is an extremely healthy squash. It is rich in zinc, copper, Vitamin B1, B2 and B6. It also contains high amount of calcium, and thus, it is one of the healthiest vegetables on Earth.

This dish is full of nutrients and colors. If you don't like to eat zucchini, try out this dish, and you will have to change your mind.

Yield: 3 - 4 persons

Total Prep Time: 25 minutes

Total Cooking Time: 40 minutes

List of Ingredients:

- Zucchini 2 medium
- Fresh tomatoes 2 diced
- Diced sweet red pepper 1 medium
- Minced garlic 3 cloves
- Skinless boneless chicken breast 2 medium (about 400gms)
- Olive oil 1 Tbsp.
- Basil dried 1 tsp.
- Oregano leaf dried ½ tsp.
- Rosemary dried ¼ tsp.
- Freshly grounded black pepper ½ tsp.
- Chicken broth (low sodium) 3 cups
- Sugar 1 tsp.
- White vinegar 1 tsp.
- Dry pasta 2 cups
- Cornstarch 1 Tbsp.

- Parmesan cheese shredded 3 Tbsp.
- Fresh parsley chopped 2 Tbsp.
- Water ½ cup

xxxxxxxxxxxxxxxxxxxxxxxxxxxxxxxxxxxxxxxxxxxx

Instructions:

1. Cut zucchini in small dice.

2. Cut sweet red pepper and tomatoes in large dice.

3. Cut chicken breasts into 1-inche pieces or bite size pieces.

4. Heat olive oil in a large pot on medium high heat.

5. Add chicken and minced garlic and sauté for approximately 10 minutes or until lightly browned.

6. Add sweet red pepper, tomatoes, and zucchini in it.

7. Sprinkle rosemary, basil, oregano and black pepper.

8. Stir and sauté vegetables for 4 to 5 minutes or until just tender crisp.

9. Remove the pot from heat.

10. In another pan heat chicken broth on medium high heat, when it starts to boil add pasta in it and stir well.

11. Cook pasta according to package direction.

12. In a small bowl add cornstarch and water and whisk until no lumps remain.

13. Put the chicken and vegetable pot again on heat add pasta with remaining liquid, sugar vinegar, and cornstarch mixture and stir and cook for 2 to 3 minutes or until sauce thickens.

14. Garnish with parmesan cheese and chopped parsley and serve.

Recipe 20: Grilled Turkey Casserole

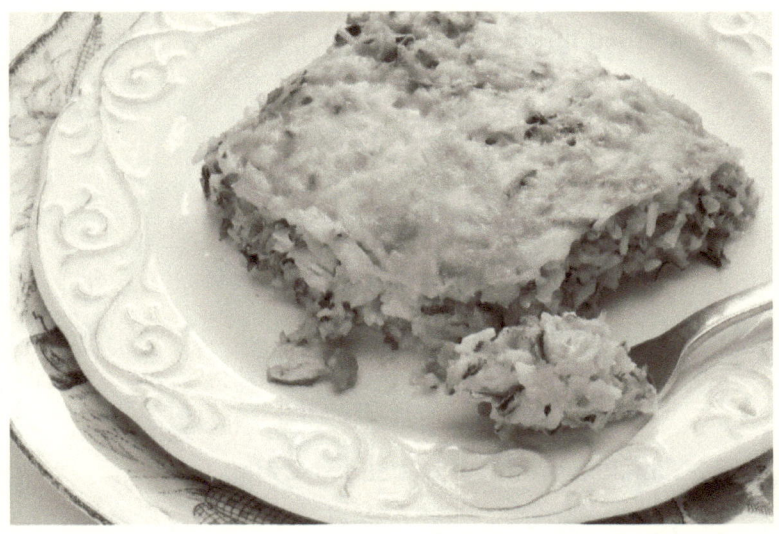

To prepare this recipe, you need to use both stove and oven. It is extremely delicious recipe with turkey in it. This could be your main course dish during family dinner, and everyone will love it. It will take some time to get ready, but it worth it. Do try it.

Yield: 5 – 6 persons

Total Prep Time: 10 minutes

Total Cooking Time: 30 minutes

List of Ingredients:

- White bread medium diced 3 cups
- Grilled turkey cut into ¾ -inch pieces 4 cups
- Canola oil ¼ cup
- Olive oil 2 Tbsp.
- Yellow onion small diced 1 small onion
- Minced garlic 2 cloves
- All-purpose flour ¼ cup
- 2% milk 1 cup
- Chicken broth (no salt added) 2 cups
- Curry powder 2 tsp.
- Broccoli florets 3 cups
- Green pepper chopped ½ cup
- Red pepper chopped ½ cup
- Grounded black pepper to taste

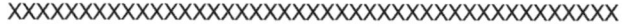

Instructions:

1. Preheat the oven to 400 degrees.

2. Heat canola oil in a medium pot over medium heat.

3. Add garlic and onion, cook for 7 minutes or until it is slightly softened (not browned).

4. Add flour while whisking continuously for 1 minute.

5. Now slowly whisk in chicken broth and milk.

6. Continue whisking until the mixture is smooth.

7. Stir sauce frequently until simmer.

8. Add curry powder and black pepper.

9. Stir in broccoli and sweet peppers and cook for 5 minutes or until beginning to soft.

10. Add grilled turkey and cook for 2 minutes.

11. Take an 8-inches square baking dish and transfer the mixture in it.

12. In another small bowl toss bread with olive oil until coated.

13. Top turkey mixture with the bread.

14. Bake until the sauce is bubbling and bread becomes golden brown. Approximately 15 minutes.

Chapter III - Low Potassium Recipes

xxxxxxxxxxxxxxxxxxxxxxxxxxxxxxxxxxxxxxxxxxxxxx

Recipe 21: Thai Fish Soup

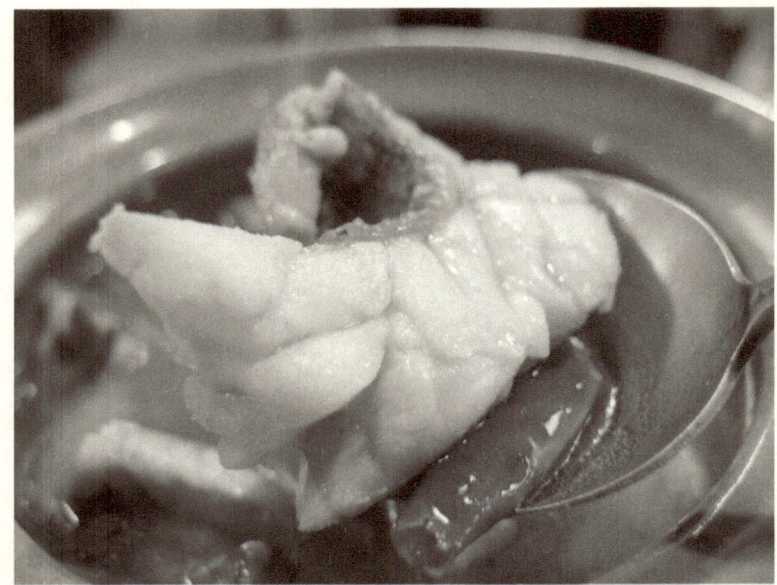

As the name is suggesting, this soup is a traditional soup of Thailand. It is made with white fish fillets (you can use either frozen or fresh). It is very tasty and nourishing. You are definitely going to love this soup.

Yield: 3 – 4

Total Prep Time: 15 minutes

Total Cooking Time: 10 minutes

List of Ingredients:

- Water 5 cups
- White fish fillets frozen 2 fillets
- Green onion chopped 1 cup
- ·Chopped garlic   2 cloves
- Minced ginger 1 Tbsp.
- Carrots diced 1 cup
- Celery diced 1 cup
- Basil to taste
- Cilantro 1 Tbsp.
- Black pepper powder ½ tsp. or to taste
- Lime juice 1 Tbsp. (juice of 1 lime)
- Bean sprouts 1 cup
- Long grain rice cooked 1 cup
- Red chili de-seeded and finely chopped 1 small
- Oil 1 Tbsp.

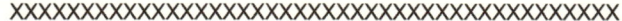

xxxxxxxxxxxxxxxxxxxxxxxxxxxxxxxxxxxxxxxxxxx

Instructions:

1. Boil water in a pan.

2. To reduce the potassium limit, in a separate pan bring carrots to boil and drain them.

3. In a pan add 1 Tbsp. oil sauté garlic, ginger, green onion, and celery over medium high heat.

4. Add boiling water, carrots, and fish.

5. Simmer until fish is cooked.

6. Add basil, cilantro, black pepper, and chopped red chili.

7. Simmer for 5 minutes.

8. Add bean sprouts and cooked rice and cook for 4 to 6 minutes.

9. Garnish with chopped cilantro and squeeze lime juice.

Recipe 22: Meatloaf Sandwiches

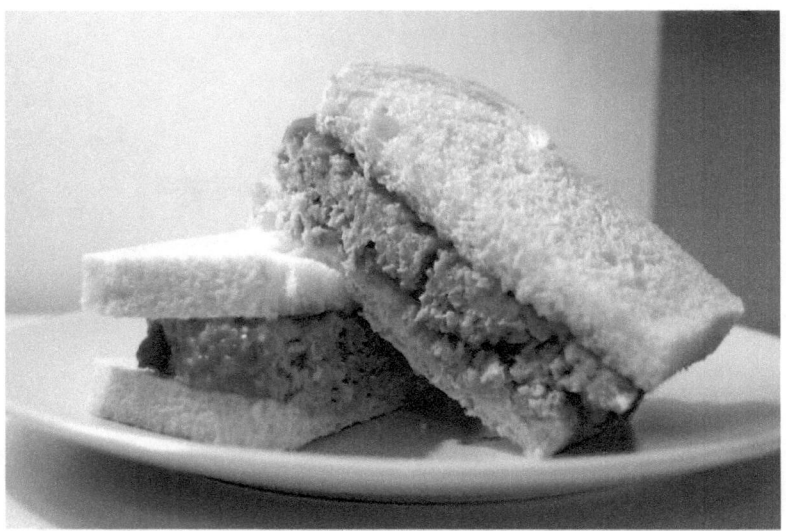

Sandwiches are a hit for every occasion. They can be consumed at breakfast, lunch, or in evening with a cup of coffee. These meatloaf sandwiches are low in potassium. In this recipe, beef is used, but you can use any other meat as well. The sandwich mixer can be stored for a couple of days in refrigerator.

Yield: 4 – 6

Total Prep Time: 25 minutes

Total Cooking Time:50 minutes

List of Ingredients:

For Meatloaf:

- Unsalted saltine-type crackers 20 squares

- Onion finely chopped 2 Tbsp.

- Lean ground beef 1 pound (10% fat)

- Egg 1 large

- 1% low fat milk 2 Tbsp.

- Black pepper grounded ¼ tsp.

- Catsup 1/3 cup

- Brown sugar 1 Tbsp.

- Apple cider vinegar ½ tsp.

- Water 1 tsp.

For Sandwiches:

- White bread slices 12 slices

- Lettuce roughly chopped 1 cup

- Onion sliced 1 large

xxxxxxxxxxxxxxxxxxxxxxxxxxxxxxxxxxxxxxxxxxx

Instructions:

1. Preheat oven to 375 F.

2. Take a large zip lock plastic bag, and place crackers in it and crush them with a rolling pin.

3. Lightly coat a loaf pan with a nonstick cooking spray.

4. In a mixing bowl, combine crushed crackers, ground beef, finely chopped onion, milk, egg, and black pepper.

5. Mix well.

6. Add this mixture to loaf pan and place it in oven.

7. Bake it for 40 minutes.

8. Mix catsup, vinegar, brown sugar, and water in a small bowl to make topping sauce.

9. Remove meatloaf after 40 minutes from the oven and cover with sauce.

10. Return meatloaf pan to the oven, and bake for 10 minutes more.

11. Remove the pan from oven, let rest it for 15 minutes before cutting into slices.

12. Slice into six thick portions.

13. Take a bread slice, and place meatloaf slice on it.

14. Top it with lettuce and sliced onion, and cover with other slice.

15. Repeat the procedure with all bread slices.

Recipe 23: Zucchini and Corn Pancakes with Chili Lime Dip

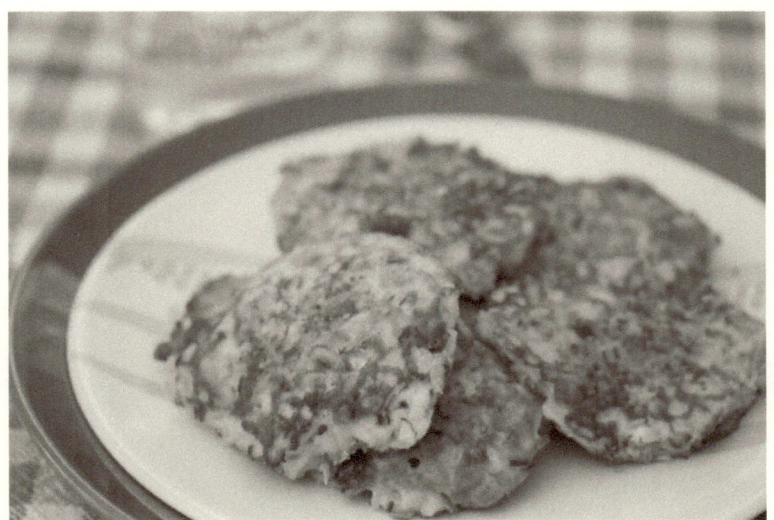

This is another healthy recipe of pancakes. If you are making these pancakes for breakfast, you can utilize them as they are. But if you want to have Zucchini and corn pancakes as evening snacks, make this finger-licking Chili Lime Dip as well.

Yield: 4 – 5

Total Prep Time: 15 minutes

Total Cooking Time: 5 minutes

Chilling Time: 30 minutes

List of Ingredients:

For pancakes:

- Zucchini shredded 2 medium
- Corn 1 cup
- Eggs 3
- White sugar 1 Tbsp.
- Vegetable oil 2 tsp.
- Milk ½ cup
- All-purpose flour 1 cup
- Baking soda 1 tsp.
- Chopped cilantro 2 Tbsp.
- Black pepper powder ½ tsp.
- Ground cumin ½ tsp.
- Cooking spray as per requirement

For chili lime dip:

- Silken tofu ½ cup
- Mayonnaise 2 Tbsp.
- Roasted red pepper from a jar ½ cup
- Chili powder 1 tsp.
- Onion powder 1 tsp.
- Lime juice 1 ½ Tbsp.
- Fresh cilantro chopped 3 Tbsp.

xxxxxxxxxxxxxxxxxxxxxxxxxxxxxxxxxxxxxxxxxxx

Instructions:

For Pancakes:

1. In a large bowl, beat eggs, and then add milk, sugar, flour, vegetable oil, and baking soda.

2. Mix well until smooth.

3. Fold in cumin, black pepper, cilantro, corn, and zucchini.

4. Warm a fry pan over medium heat.

5. Coat it with cooking spray.

6. Spoon ¼ cup batter into fry pan.

7. Flip only one time, cook until golden on both sides.

8. Serve hot with chili lime dip.

For Chili lime dip:

1. Take a blender add all the ingredients in it and blend for 30 seconds or until smooth.

2. In a small bowl transfer the ingredients of the blender.

3. Cover and refrigerate for 30 minutes.

Recipe 24: Chicken with Pineapple and Honey

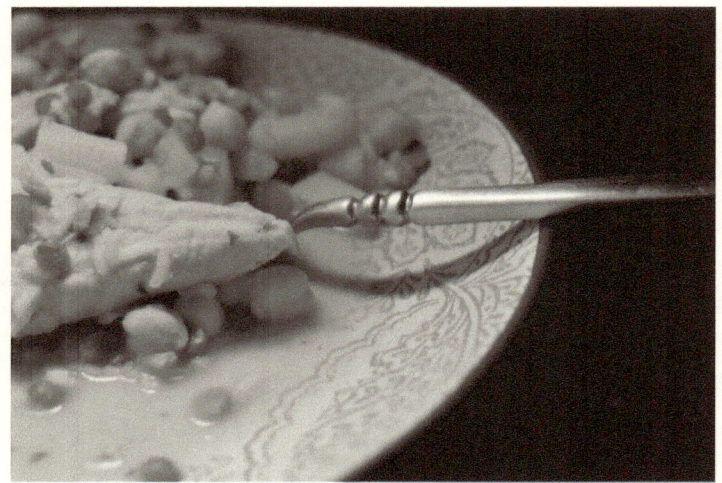

This low potassium chicken dish is super easy to make. The preparation and cooking time is not even an hour. Almost all ingredients are available in our kitchens, so whenever you think, you want something juicy and tasty, prepare this dish. Eating it with rice will be feel you full, and it could be your main dish for dinner or even lunch.

Yield: 3 – 4

Total Prep Time: 10 minutes

Total Cooking Time: 40 minutes

List of Ingredients:

- Pineapple slices canned, in juice 20 ounces
- Chicken breast skinless boneless 1 pound
- Minced garlic 2 cloves
- Ground thyme 1 tsp.
- Black pepper powder ¼ tsp.
- Vegetable oil 1 Tbsp.
- Corn starch 1 Tbsp.
- Honey 3 Tbsp.
- Dijon mustard 3 Tbsp.
- White rice cooked 2 cups
- Water 2 Tbsp.

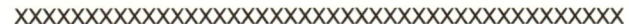

xxxxxxxxxxxxxxxxxxxxxxxxxxxxxxxxxxxxxxxxxx

Instructions:

1. Drain pineapples from juice and reserve the juice.

2. Rub thyme and garlic on chicken and sprinkle black pepper.

3. In a nonstick skillet or wok, heat oil over high heat.

4. Add chicken and cook until brown from both sides.

5. Reduce heat to medium, add Dijon mustard, pineapple juice, and honey.

6. Stir and spoon sauce over chicken.

7. Cover and simmer for 10 minutes.

8. In a small bowl, combine 2 Tbsp. of water with corn starch and add to chicken and sauce.

9. Now add pineapple slices keep stirring.

10. Cook until the sauce boil and thickens.

11. Serve with rice.

Recipe 25: Glazed Chicken Wings

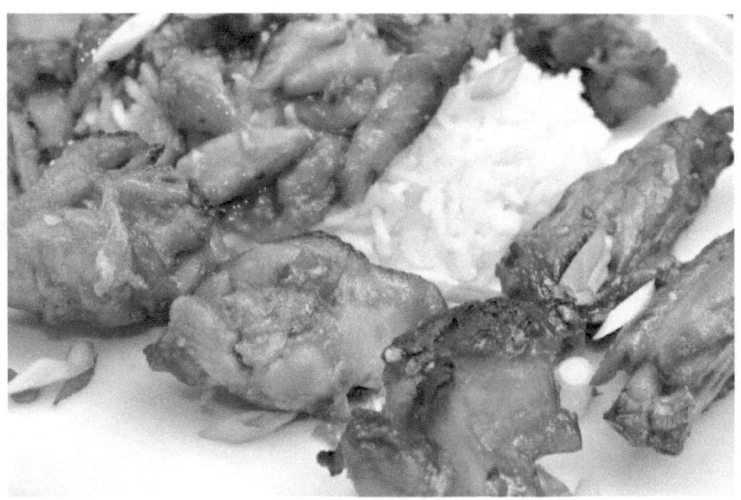

This recipe of delicious and mouth-watering chicken wings is simply amazing. It is easy to make and contains low potassium content. You can marinade and store the wings for future use as well. Make sure chicken is marinated for at-least 7 hours, so the spices can penetrate in the wings. You can use a dip to double the joy of Glazed Chicken Wings.

Yield: 6 – 7

Total Prep Time: 15 minutes

Total Cooking Time: 1 hour

List of Ingredients:

- Chicken wings 7 pounds (36 wings)
- Green onion chopped 4 medium
- Reduced sodium soya sauce 2 Tbsp.
- Honey ¼ cup
- Granulated sugar 2 Tbsp.
- Brown sugar ¼ cup
- All spice powder 2 tsp.
- Hot sauce 2 tsp.
- Dried thyme 2 tsp.
- Ginger chopped 1 tsp.
- Minced garlic 1 tsp.
- Apple cider vinegar ¼ cup
- Lime juice ¼ cup
- Cranberry juice ¼ cup

xxxxxxxxxxxxxxxxxxxxxxxxxxxxxxxxxxxxxxxxxxxx

Instructions:

1. In a large mixing bowl, add green onion, soya sauce, honey, granulated sugar, brown sugar, all spice powder, hot sauce, dried thyme, ginger, garlic, apple cider vinegar, lime juice, and cranberry juice.

2. Mix well all the ingredients to make a marinade.

3. Reserve ¾ cup of marinade for glaze.

4. Take a large re-sealable plastic bag or container and place all chicken wings in it.

5. Pour the marinade over wings.

6. Cover and marinate.

7. Keep in refrigerator for 6 to 8 hours.

8. Preheat oven to 375 F.

9. On a baking sheet place all chicken wings.

10. Bake for 20 minutes.

11. To prepare glaze take a small saucepan and add reserved ¾ cup marinade in it.

12. Bring it to boil.

13. Cook on medium low flame for 10 minutes or until it thickens slightly to a glaze.

14. Remove chicken wings from oven after 20 minutes and brush all the wings with the glaze.

15. Raise your oven temperature to 400 F.

16. Place chicken wings in oven and cook about another 20 minutes or until done.

17. Garnish with chopped green onion and serve.

Recipe 26: Cucumber and Dill Cool Soup

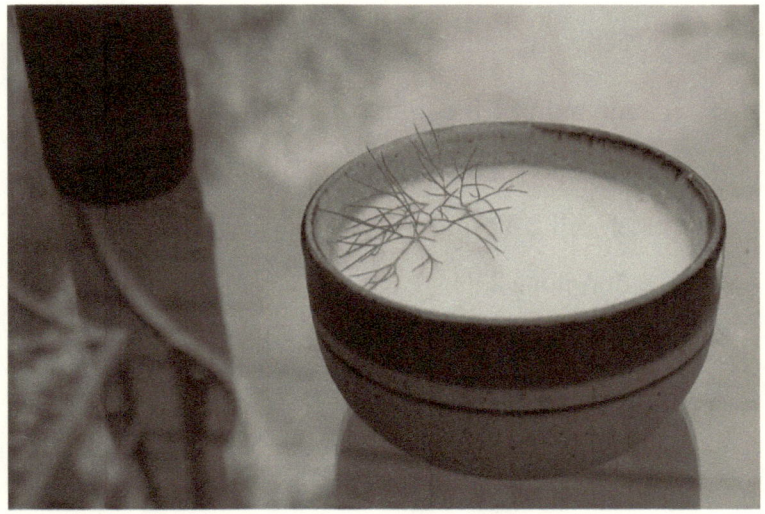

This recipe will give you an end result of a mouth-watering soup. It's very tasty and healthy soup. This soup is especially beneficial for summers, as cucumber helps you in keeping yourself hydrated. Cucumber has many other benefits too; it helps in weight loss, provides vitamins, decrease risk of cancer, to name a few.

Yield: 2 – 3

Total Prep Time: 15 minutes

Chilling Time: 1 hour

List of Ingredients:

- Cucumbers 2 medium
- Sweet white onion 1/3 cup
- Green onion 1 medium
- Fresh mint leaves ¼ cup
- Fresh dill 2 Tbsp.
- Lemon juice 2 Tbsp.
- Water 2/3 cup
- Half and half cream ½ cup
- Sour cream 1/3 cup
- Pepper ½ tsp.
- Fresh dill sprigs for garnish as per requirement

xxxxxxxxxxxxxxxxxxxxxxxxxxxxxxxxxxxxxxxxxxxxxx

Instructions:

1. Peel and remove the seeds from cucumber, and cut them into small cubes.

2. Chop mint leaves, sweet onion, and dill.

3. Place cucumber, dill, mint, onion, green onion, lemon juice, water, half and half cream, sour cream, and pepper in blender.

4. Blend well until smooth.

5. Cover and keep it in refrigerator for 4 hours or until chilled.

6. Garnish this yummy cool soup with dill sprigs and serve.

7. You can serve it with tuna salad, chicken salad, or egg salad sandwich.

Recipe 27: Eggplant and Bell Pepper Casserole

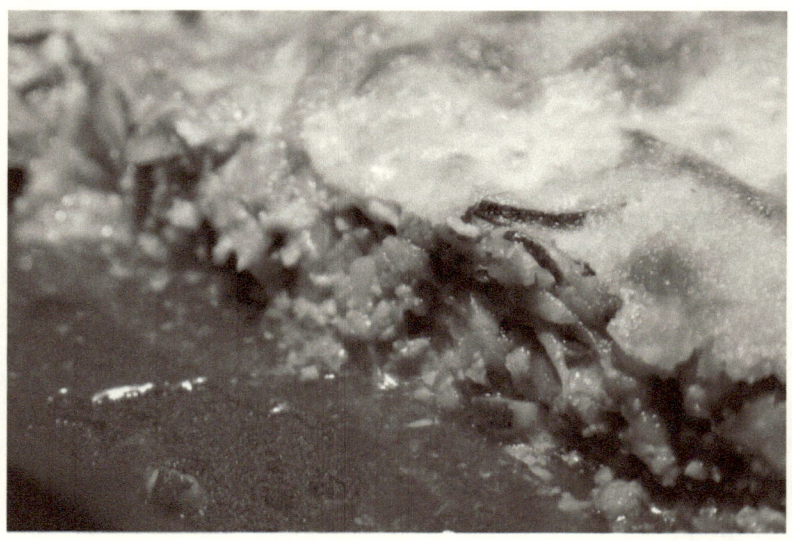

Casserole is basically a French word used for large deep pans. Any food which is cooked and served in a casserole, is also known as casserole. In this recipe, eggplant and bell pepper are cooked in such a pan, as the name suggests. It is a fulling and tasty dish. You can have it in Lunch, or use as a side dish for parties.

Yield: 2 – 3

Total Prep Time: 15 minutes

Total Cooking Time: 40 minutes

List of Ingredients:

- Eggplant 2 medium
- Olive oil 1 Tbsp.
- ·Butter ¼ cup
- Onion ½ cup
- Green bell pepper ¼ cup
- Garlic 5 cloves
- Cayenne paper ½ tsp.
- Black pepper ½ tsp.
- Ground thyme ½ tsp.
- Egg 1 large
- Plain bread crumbs ½ cup

xxxxxxxxxxxxxxxxxxxxxxxxxxxxxxxxxxxxxxxxxx

Instructions:

1. Preheat oven to 350 F.

2. Cut eggplants into cubes.

3. Chop garlic finely.

4. Chop bell pepper and onion.

5. Beat egg in a separate bowl.

6. Heat butter and oil in a large skillet over medium heat.

7. Sauté onion, garlic, and green pepper in heated oil.

8. Add in black pepper and cayenne pepper, and sauté for a while.

9. Add eggplant and thyme and cook until eggplant softens.

10. Stir often.

11. Keep 2 Tbsp. of bread crumbs for topping.

12. Add the remaining bread crumbs to eggplant.

13. Cook for 15 minutes.

14. By stirring quickly, add the beaten egg to the mixture so egg does not solidify.

15. Place in a casserole dish.

16. Sprinkle remaining bread crumbs.

17. Bake for 25 minutes.

18. Cool on rack and serve.

19. You can freeze or refrigerate leftover casserole.

Recipe 28: Apple Pie

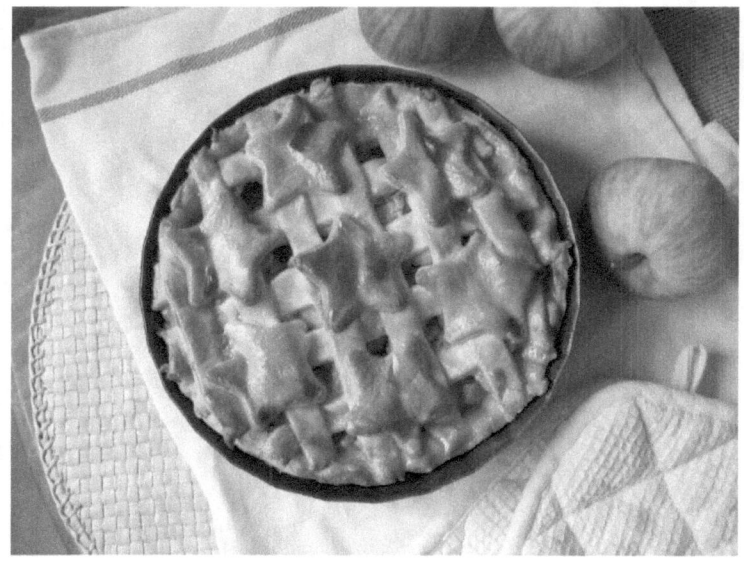

Apple pie is sort of fruit tart, which is famous all around the world, especially in the USA. It is loved equally by people of all ages. On some occasions, apple pie is served with ice-cream, whipped cream, or cheddar cheese. It's a low potassium sweet dish. If you haven't try this recipe yet, go and start preparations for it.

Yield: 5 – 6

Total Prep Time: 1 hour

Total Cooking Time: 45 minutes

List of Ingredients:

- Apples 6 medium
- Granulated sugar ½ cup
- Cinnamon powder 1 tsp.
- Butter 6 Tbsp.
- All-purpose flour 2 to 2/3 cups
- Shortening 1 cup
- Water 6 Tbsp.

xxxxxxxxxxxxxxxxxxxxxxxxxxxxxxxxxxxxxxxxxx

Instructions:

1. Heat up oven to 400 F.

2. Peel all apples, core them, and cut into slightly thin slices.

3. In a large bowl, put apple slices, and add cinnamon powder, and sugar in it.

4. Mix all the ingredients carefully, so that all apple slices are covered with cinnamon powder, and sugar.

5. Now cover that bowl, and put it aside.

6. Take another large bowl, put flour in it. With the help of a pastry blender, carefully mix shortening with flour.

7. Add chilled water to the mixture slowly, only one Tbsp. at a time.

8. With the help of your hands, knead the dough, until it forms a ball.

9. Divide the dough in two equal portions.

10. Using a rolling pin, roll one portion of the kneaded dough. You can use dry flour, if required.

11. Place this rolled dough in inch pie pan (9 inch pan will do).

12. Stir cinnamon and apple mixture, and pour it in the pie pan.

13. With the help of a Tbsp., disperse butter evenly all around the pie filling.

14. After dispersing butter evenly, roll the remaining ball of dough.

15. Place this rolled dough on top of the apple filling in the pie pan.

16. Before moving to next step, make sure that apple filling is covered with the second rolled dough.

17. With the help of a sharp knife, make 4 1-inch cuts on the upper rolled dough of the apple pie. These cuts will help air to escape out while baking.

18. Before putting it in oven for baking, refrigerate the pie pan for at-least 15 minutes.

19. Place pie pan on jellyroll pan in oven in order to catch juice from pie in baking process.

20. Bake until pie crust turns to golden brown (45-60 minutes).

21. Cool on a rack before serving.

Recipe 29: Minced Beef Samosa

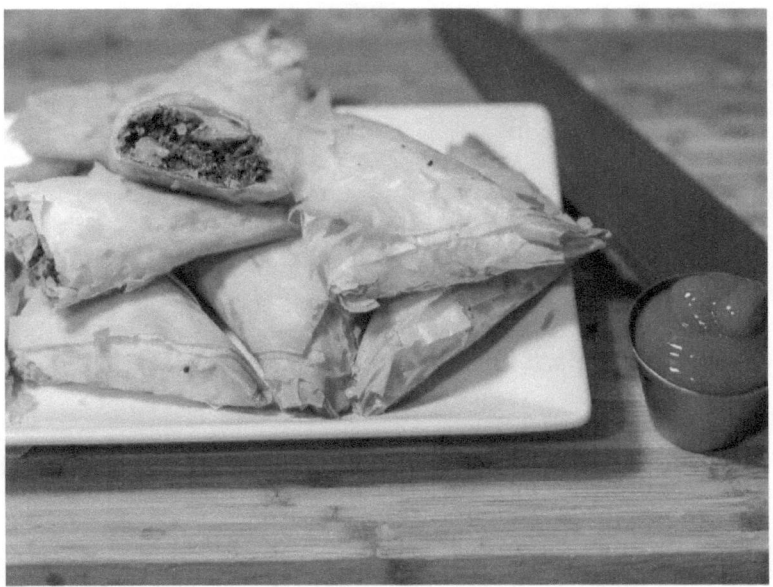

Samosa is a traditional recipe of South India. It is usually served as a side dish, or an evening snack. This is a very easy recipe of samosa that you can prepare at home. If you don't like peas, you can omit them. Serve hot samosa with tea or coffee.

Yield: 8 – 10

Total Prep Time: 25 minutes

Total Cooking Time: 20 minutes

List of Ingredients:

- Minced beef 1 pound
- Onion ¼ cup
- Ginger root 1 tsp.
- Garlic 1 clove
- Cilantro 2 Tbsp.
- Green peas (fresh) ½ cup
- Canola oil 3 Tbsp.
- Coriander powder 1 Tbsp.
- Turmeric powder ½ tsp.
- Pepper ¼ tsp.
- Lemon juice 1 tsp.
- All spice powder 1 tsp.
- Samosa pastries 24 pastries
- ·Flour 2 Tbsp.
- Water 1 ½ Tbsp.

XXXXXXXXXXXXXXXXXXXXXXXXXXXXXXXXXXXXXXXXXX

Instructions:

1. Chop ginger, garlic, and cilantro finely.

2. Chop onion finely, and set aside.

3. Take large sauce pan and heat 3 Tbsp. oil.

4. Add garlic, ginger and onion and sauté for 2 to 3 minutes.

5. Add coriander powder, turmeric powder, and cayenne pepper stir for one minute.

6. Add ground beef and all spice powder and until beef is cooked.

7. Drain excessive fat from beef mixture.

8. Include green peas and cook mixture to dry

9. Top with lemon juice and cilantro and evenly stir.

10. In a small bowl, make a thin paste with 1 tbsp. of flour and enough water.

11. Spread remaining flour on a board and roll out pastry on it.

12. In the center of the pastry, put 2 tbsp. of the beef mixture and fold diagonally to make a triangular shape.

13. Close edges with water and flour paste.

14. Repeat the procedure with all pastries.

15. Heat oil over high flame to deep fry pastries.

16. Deep fry until light golden brown.

17. To reduce fat, you can also bake the samosa on a greased baking tray for 15 minutes each side.

Recipe 30: Strawberry Jelly Stuffed French Toast

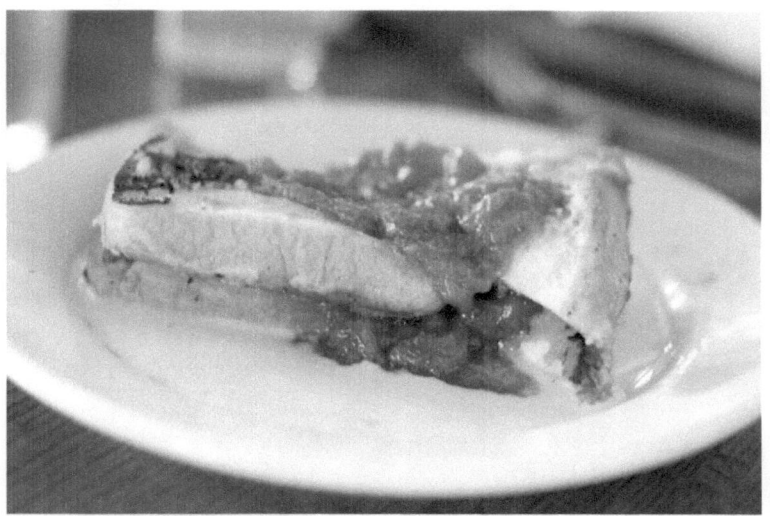

If you are thinking what to make for evening snack, here is a tasty recipe for you. It's easy to make, and you don't need too many ingredients for this recipe of French toast. If you don't have strawberry jelly, you can use any other flavored jelly.

Yield: 5 – 6

Total Prep Time: 25 minutes

Total Cooking Time: 1 hour

List of Ingredients:

- Cream cheese 8 ounces
- Loaf of day old French bread 1 pound
- Strawberry jelly 8 Tbsp.
- Eggs 6 large
- 1% low fat milk 1 cup
- Vanilla extract   1 tsp.

xxxxxxxxxxxxxxxxxxxxxxxxxxxxxxxxxxxxxxxxxxx

Instructions:

1. Slice the French bread loaf into 16 slices.

2. Bring cream cheese to room temperature, spread 1 Tbsp. on each slice of bread.

3. Top it with 1 Tbsp. strawberry jelly. Spread evenly.

4. Add other bread slice to make a sandwich.

5. Repeat the procedure until eight sandwiches are ready.

6. Take a 9"x 13" baking dish; spray it with nonstick cooking spray.

7. Place all the sandwiches in baking dish.

8. In a mixing bowl, beat eggs.

9. Add milk and vanilla extract and whisk the mixture well.

10. Pour the egg mixture over bread sandwiches.

11. Turn each sandwich to coat the slices evenly.

12. Cover and keep it in refrigerator for overnight or for at-least 8 to 12 hours.

13. Preheat your oven to 359 F.

14. Cover the sandwich pan with aluminum foil.

15. Bake for one hour or 55 minutes.

16. Take out the baking dish from oven and remove the foil, and put the dish back to give a nice golden color to the sandwiches.

17. Let it cool.

18. Garnish with strawberry slices and dust with powdered sugar.

Chapter IV - Tips to Keep Your Kidneys Healthy

Kidneys are vital organs of our body. But due to several reasons, cases of kidney disease are increasing day by day. If you have high blood pressure, diabetes, or a family history of renal problem, you are at high risk of kidney disease. Even if you don't have any of these problems, you should take care of your kidneys. Following are few tips that will help you in maintaining good kidney health:

Appropriate Intake of Water – Usually it is believed that drinking too much water can help your kidneys function properly, but no studies have proven this fact yet. No doubt that appropriate intake of water keeps you hydrated and helps your kidneys work properly, but good kidney function has nothing to do with drinking lots of water.

Stay Active and Exercise Regularly – Staying active and taking exercise regularly helps you in getting rid of extra weight, regulating your blood pressure, and thus, decreasing the chances of Chronic Kidney Disease. It is a good idea to exercise if you are healthy, but if you have some health issues, you should consult your physician to know how much exercise you can do. This is because, if you do over-exercise with certain health issues, you can put strain over your kidneys.

Take Healthy Diet – Healthy eating habits can prevent you from many health conditions that lead to Chronic Kidney Disease. Avoid restaurant and processed food as much as you can. Limit your salt intake, and for this purpose, it is best to prepare your own food, so you can control the amount of salt added in the food. Moderate eating habits not only help you in controlling your weight, but also regulates your blood pressure.

Quit Smoking Today – With many other problems, smoking can cause kidney problems in your body as well. Chemicals released in body due to smoking damage blood vessels, which results in decreased blood flow towards your kidneys. Without adequate amount of blood, kidneys cannot deliver their best. Smoking also increases the risk of blood pressure, and kidney cancer chances are also increased by 50%.

Keep Blood Sugar Level in Control – Diabetes or high blood sugar level adversely affect your kidneys. If you have diabetes, it is important to check it regularly, and keep it under control.

Regulate your Blood Pressure – You all may know that high blood pressure leads to heart attack, stroke, or other heart diseases, but most of you don't know that it is one of the most common cause of kidney damage. You should keep your blood pressure regularly checked, and controlled. It is likely to cause more kidney damage, when associated with high cholesterol, Cardio-Vascular Disease, and diabetes.

Limited Use of Over the Counter Medication – If taken regularly or for prolonged period of time, many commonly used drugs can cause kidney damage. If you have normal working, healthy kidneys, you won't be risked by the use of these medicines. But regular use of these medicines for any chronic pain, can cause severe kidney damage. You should not use them too often, and consult your physician to find another way to get rid of your pain.

With any Risk Factor, Keep Kidney Function Screened –

If you have many or any of the certain risk factors, you should keep an eye on your kidney function. Some of these factors are:

- Diabetes
- High blood pressure
- Obesity
- Renal family history

About the Author

Heston Brown is an accomplished chef and successful e-book author from Palo Alto California. After studying cooking at The New England Culinary Institute, Heston stopped briefly in Chicago where he was offered head chef at some of the city's most prestigious restaurants. Brown decide that he missed the rolling hills and sunny weather of California and moved back to his home state to open up his own catering company and give private cooking classes.

Heston lives in California with his beautiful wife of 18 years and his two daughters who also have aspirations to follow in their father's footsteps and pursue careers in the culinary arts. Brown is well known for his delicious fish and chicken dishes and teaches these recipes as well as many others to his students.

When Heston gave up his successful chef position in Chicago and moved back to California, a friend suggested he use the internet to share his recipes with the world and so he did! To date, Heston Brown has written over 1000 e-books that contain recipes, cooking tips, business strategies for catering companies and a self-help book he wrote from personal experience.

He claims his wife has been his inspiration throughout many of his endeavours and continues to be his partner in business as well as life. His greatest joy is having all three women in his life in the kitchen with him cooking their favourite meal while his favourite jazz music plays in the background.

Author's Afterthoughts

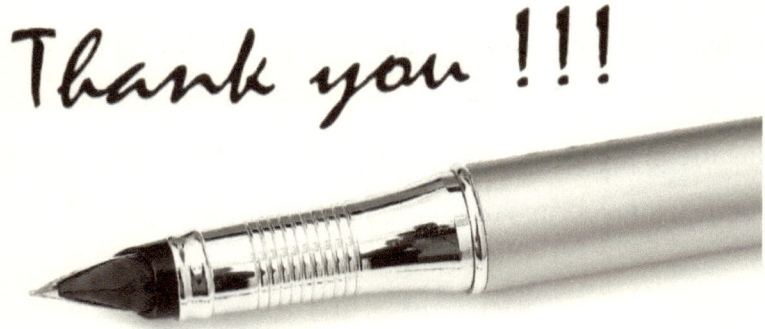

Thank you to all the readers who invested time and money into my book! I cherish every one of you and hope you took the same pleasure in reading it as I did in writing it.

Out of all of the books out there, you chose mine and for that I am truly grateful. It makes the effort worth it when I know my readers are enjoying my work from beginning to end.

Please take a few minutes to write an Amazon review so that others can benefit from your opinions and insight. Your review will help countless other readers make an informed choice

Thank you so much,

Heston Brown